Living out

GOD'S PURPOSE

in our senior years

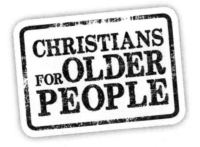

CHRISTIANS
FOR OLDER
PEOPLE

Living out

GOD'S PURPOSE

in our senior years

Developing Usefulness in Old Age

Louise Morse & Roger Hitchings

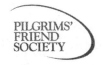

PILGRIMS'
FRIEND
SOCIETY

Living out God's Purpose in our Senior Years

Developing usefulness in old age.

Copyright July 2014 The Pilgrims' Friend Society.

A catalogue record for this publication is available from the British Library

ISBN: 978-0-9930148-3-3

Designed and typeset by: Pete Barnsley (Creativehoot.com)

Printed and bound by CPI Group (UK) Ltd, Croydon, CR0 4YY

First published in the UK in 2014 by the Pilgrims' Friend Society

175 Tower Bridge Road, London SE1 2AL.
Tel +44 0300 303 1400

Email: info@pilgrimsfriend.org.uk
Website: www.pilgrimsfriend.org.uk

Distributed by the Pilgrims' Friend Society.

ABOUT THE AUTHORS

Louise Morse is Media and Communications Manager with the Pilgrims' Friend Society. She is also a Cognitive Behavioural Therapist, with a Master's dissertation that examined the effect on families of caring for a relative with dementia.

She is author of books on dementia: *Could it be Dementia? – Losing your mind doesn't mean losing your soul*; *Dementia: Frank and Linda's Story – New Understanding, New Approaches, New Hope, and Worshipping with Dementia*, published by Lion Monarch. A new book, *Dementia: Pathways to Hope* is due in November and a loose-leaf information pack, *Helping to put the Pieces Together*, is published by the Pilgrims' Friend Society. She is a regular contributor to the Christian press.

Louise is also a speaker at national and regional conferences. She continually researches issues of old age, and is passionate about attitudes and decisions that affect older people. She brings a Christian perspective to all her work. She is on Facebook and Twitter, and runs a blog: blog.pilgrimsfriend.org.uk

Roger Hitchings is a speaker and writer on issues affecting older people, particularly from a Biblical perspective. In writing *Could it be Dementia?* Louise drew extensively from a body of Roger's work in the form of transcripts of talks he had given at different times.

Roger worked in a professional capacity with older people for 25 years and then for 15 years as a Pastor of an independent evangelical church in the East Midlands until his retirement in 2012. He believes strongly that the church is strengthened when older people are encouraged and enabled to function as the Bible teaches they ought to be, and that even in dementia Christians serve God.

CONTENTS

Step 3 – Recognising the hindrances and the helps

Step 4 – The Key to Usefulness

Empowering and Engaging Older People 31

UNDERSTANDING THE DIFFERENT VIEWS OF OLD AGE

What do we mean by old age?

Each year we attend a national Christian event which takes place over two weeks in the summer time. It is attended by around 30,000 people, and many of them are families with children. In the course of each day there are activities for each age range. One year we took part in a competition for the children. The aim was to keep them engaged and to give them an idea of the work of each organisation that had a stand in the market place. The children visited every organisation and those participating either gave them tasks to do or gave them questions to answer.

When they came to our stand, cards clutched in their hands and all expectant, our questions were, 'When does a person become old?', 'Are there older people in your church?' and 'How does your church look after them?'

The most interesting thing to see was how their responses mirrored those of adults. Our view of what constitutes old age depends on our age at the time we're thinking about it. To a six year old a fifteen year old was quite old, and to a fifteen year old, twenty-five was 'knocking on a bit'. We asked a group of three children who were standing in front of their father, 'At what age is someone old?' and their father whispered over their heads, 'I hope they don't give mine!'

After our seminar on 'Preparing for a Great Old Age', a participant came to our stand and said, 'I thought I was old and past it. I'm seventy, a retired teacher. But after listening to you I realise I have plenty of years ahead of me. I'm not on the rubbish heap!'

More and more people are living into their nineties, and even hundreds. And there is good news and bad news, but there is more good news than bad. Cases of dementia continue to increase and there is still no cure. On the other hand, a Cambridge study has shown that the prevalence of dementia is much lower than predicted in the 1990s, and the incidence is reducing. And recently, the prestigious Mayo Clinic published findings of a study showing that in cases of mild cognitive impairment (MCI) in older people, more people reverted to normal than went on to develop dementia.

Stories abound of older people achieving great things. For example, the 87 year old lady who lost her sight quite suddenly, but went on to use the disability as a means of winning a number of people to Christ, asking them to read some Christian tracts to her as they waited at a bus stop; the 93 year old lady who came out of retirement for the third time to advise a design firm on what was best for older people; the gentleman who became the first to complete a marathon at the age of 100; the 94 year old who won accolades for a lecture in his specialism in Berlin, and Diane 93, one of our supporters, who was asked to take Bible studies in the care home she moved into.

The front cover photograph is of Ruth Edwards, former home matron who served on PFS committees and was a vigorous supporter until her late eighties.

Old age is not what it used to be. People are

not only living longer but generally speaking, living 'better', too.

The Bible tells us to 'number our days,' (Psalm 90:12.) It doesn't mean that we need to count them off, but that we should make our days count. Another, similar instruction is in Ephesians 5:16, to *'redeem the days, because they are evil,'* – to bring good things into our days to overcome the darkness.

In this booklet we look at how we can make our days count all the days of our lives, and the things that can prevent us as we grow older.

How the world sees old age

Society judges people on three values: the first is on their physical and intellectual abilities, the second on their function in life and how well they do it, and the third on their relationships.

Ageism is endemic in the UK, with older people being judged as having no value as they are not seen as contributors to society. Their charitable work, and their support for their families and churches is usually overlooked. On the contrary, the perception is that they are a drain, a demand on both the State's and their families' resources. Economists have said that because they purchase less than younger generations, older people are slowing growth in the global economy. Thinking like this reflects how globalisation, driven by commercial interests, is digging ever more deeply into our cultural ethics, reducing the value of human beings to figures on a balance sheet. The result is a secular mind-set that sees older people as 'takers' instead of 'contributors'.

The danger is that this view can be unconsciously absorbed by older Christians and influence not only their individual attitudes, but that of the church. This is often exacerbated by the youth culture of many churches where older people are seen as secondary to the main aim and objective. The world, the church and older people themselves often combine to diminish their value. Despite a growing number of older people very few churches only have pastoral workers for the young. But this is not how God has designed old age, nor how He sees it.

How God sees old age

Old age is not a mistake in God's design. He planned old age to be a season of harvest for His older people, a time of accumulated wisdom and experience from a life spent with Him. It is also a time of continuing growth. *'They will still yield fruit in old age; they shall be full of sap and very green,'* Psalm 92:14

Older believers are repositories of God's goodness over the years. They are full of accounts of His acts in their lives. Many of the psalms say these should be shared with others, to give God glory, and to encourage and build up the others. (Psalm 78 is an example.)

Older people should be respected for their wisdom: Leviticus 19:32. In an ancient culture there was a saying that the ruler did not worry until the grey beards murmured.

John's letter to the church shows the balance of young and old: *'I am writing to you, fathers, because you know Him who has been from the beginning. I am writing to you, young men, because you have overcome the evil one. I have written to you, children, because you know the Father,'* 1 John 2: 12-14.

The same model is seen in Titus 2:1-4. *'You, however, must teach what is appropriate to sound doctrine. Teach the older men to be temperate, worthy of respect, self-controlled, and sound in faith, in love and in endurance. 'Likewise, teach the older women to be reverent in the way they live, not to be slanderers or addicted to much wine, but to teach what is good. Then they can urge the younger women to love their husbands and children.'*

Many things can only be learnt by experience, and experience is something that comes with years. Clearly, the young and the old provide a balance in the church.

'The glory of young men is their strength, but the splendour of old men is their grey hair,' Proverbs 20:29. Grey hair is a synonym for wisdom.

Old age is something that God meant to be enjoyed. Old age is:

- a blessing

- a time of fullness in knowing God

- to be a period of growth

- to be marked by a particular religious and ethical witness and testimony

- a time of exhibiting the fruit of the Spirit
  – *'love, joy, peace, patience, kindness, goodness, faithfulness, gentleness and self-control.'* Galatians 5:22,23

- a time for sharing God's goodness manifested over a life time

- a time given to us by the Lord to fully prove His grace and to prepare ourselves to enter glory satisfied with all God's goodness. Psalm 91:16

- a time for mentoring the younger generation.

STEP 2

UNDERSTANDING WHAT WE MEAN BY BEING USEFUL

What do we mean by being useful?

Being 'useful' means different things to different people. Often 'being useful' is linked to the roles we have in our lives. When these roles change – for instance, when work is left behind in retirement, or children grow up and leave home there can be a sense of our having lost our usefulness.

Usefulness means more than 'doing', however good those activities may be. It can be satisfying to feel a sense of achievement from things we accomplish. We believe that in God's eyes usefulness means accomplishing His purposes in the world, and that can mean in big things and in little. We are told to encourage one another, for example, and a word of encouragement can take less than a minute but can have a resonance that lasts a lifetime.

As Christians, our usefulness is much wider and deeper than our career, or even being a parent. It was planned for each one of us before we were born and extends beyond our death into eternity.

The Scriptures tell us that we are here by design, and for a purpose. Ephesians 2:10 says: *'For we are His workmanship, created in Christ Jesus for good works, which God prepared beforehand that we should walk in them.'*

There is great assurance in the verse, because it tells us that God has not only equipped us to do 'good works', but has laid them out ahead of us. We don't have to go looking for them. And we are to do them whole-heartedly.

Our definition of 'usefulness', therefore, is doing the 'good works' God brings to you. There will be different 'good works' depending on the talents and gifts that He has given to each person. Exodus 35 is a good example of those He had given to individuals for the building of the Tabernacle, and Ephesians 4: 11-13 show different roles for building up the church. 1 Peter 4:10; Romans 12:16, and Ephesians 4:7 urge us to use our gifts both in the church and in reaching others around us. And of course, Solomon urges us, 'Whatever your right hand finds to do, do it with all your strength,' Ecclesiastes 9:10

You might find it helpful to write a list of all the ways in which you are 'useful'. Write them all down, big and small. Then read them. You will be surprised at how God is working His purpose out in your life, for you and through you.

Spiritual prosperity in later years

Psalm 92 gives us an encouraging picture of spiritual prosperity in later years. It is the expression of older persons' character and intrinsic value.

1. Older people have gained wisdom

2 Corinthians 1: 3-5 tells of experience and wisdom gained.

2. Older people have things to share

'O God, from my youth you have taught me, and I still proclaim your wondrous deeds.'

—Psalm 71:8

3. Older people have proved the truth of biblical precepts

'I have been young, and now am old, yet I

have not seen the righteous forsaken or his
children begging for bread.'

—Psalm 37:25

4. Older people have learnt patience, and understand God's time span

'But do not overlook this one fact, beloved,
that with the Lord one day is as a thousand
years, and a thousand years as one day,'

—1 Peter 3:8

5. Older people understand the importance of personal, spiritual growth, and with physical frailty they appreciate the importance of 'being', as opposed to 'doing,' and welcome the days of growing closer to Him. This time of 'being' can be a time of great spiritual growth and deep intercession.

'My soul longs, yes faints for the courts of
the Lord; my heart and flesh sing for joy to
the living God.'

—Psalm 84:1,2

6. Older people anticipate Heaven

'So we do not lose heart. Though our outer self
is wasting away, our inner self is being renewed

day by day. For this light momentary affliction is preparing for us an eternal weight of glory beyond all comparison, as we look not to the things that are seen but to the things that are unseen. For the things that are seen are transient, but the things that are unseen are eternal.'

—2 Corinthians 4: 16-18

These five categories cover the spiritual life of the older person. Spiritual life needs to be nurtured and encouraged throughout life, but especially in old age.

Telling of God's grace and goodness

Imagine how many times older people have witnessed God's grace and love throughout the years; and imagine now how much it would encourage and bless others – both believers and non-believers – if they were to share those experiences.

Being testaments of God's grace, bringing testimony of His love, is a powerful blessing which old people can and should bestow. Churches can enable this by inviting older members to give their testimony, or tell of their experiences during their lives.

'I will come and proclaim your mighty acts,
Sovereign Lord;

13

I will proclaim your righteous deeds, yours alone.
Since my youth, God, you have taught me
and to this day I declare your marvelous deeds.
Even when I am old and grey, do not forsake
me, my God,
till I declare your power to the next generation,
your mighty acts to all who are to come.'

—Psalm 71: 16-18

'He established a testimony in Jacob
and appointed a law in Israel,
which he commanded our father
to teach to their children
that the next generation might know them,
the children yet unborn,
and arise and tell them to their children,
so that they should set their hope in God
and not forget the works of God
but keep his commandments;.'

—Psalm 78: 5-7

'Give ear, O my people, to my teaching;
incline your ears to the words of my mouth!
I will open my mouth in a parable;
I will utter dark sayings from of old
things that we have heard and known,

> *that our fathers have told us.*
> *We will not hide them from their children,*
> *but tell to the coming generation*
> *the glorious deeds of the LORD, and his might,*
> *and the wonders that he has done.'*
>
> **—Psalm 78:1-4**

Exemplifying grace in daily living

'Actions speak louder than words' – One very simple and effective way that older people can be a huge blessing, especially to the younger generation, is to be an example of Jesus' grace in their day-to-day living. Seeing someone with a godly lifestyle, full of God's love and grace, is as powerful a testimony of His love as a spoken word.

> *'Remember your leaders, who spoke the word of God to you. Consider the outcome of their way of life and imitate their faith.'*
>
> **—Hebrews 13:7**

Displaying heavenly-mindedness in times of trial

In times of trouble, people tend to look to the

15

older generation for help; for their wisdom and guidance. Offering re-assurance and reminding them to bring everything to God is an invaluable service, and of course, not without Heavenly reward.

'Therefore we do not lose heart. Though outwardly we are wasting away, yet inwardly we are being renewed day by day.'

—2 Corinthians 4:16-5:5

'I have fought the good fight, I have finished the race, I have kept the faith. Now there is in store for me the crown of righteousness.'

—2 Timothy 4:7-8

Showing the power of prayer

In the movie 'Fiddler on the Roof', Tevye sang: 'If I were a rich man, I'd have the time that I lack to sit in the synagogue and pray.' What a wonderful, powerful way to spend time! In Luke 2:37 we hear of Anna, who *'… was a widow until she was eighty-four. She never left the temple but worshipped night and day, fasting and praying.'*

Younger people need the prayers of the older generation. Today's hectic pace of life means that many of the younger generation don't have the time to devote themselves in daily prayer as much as they should. Technology means that one can never truly escape the office, and the rising cost of living often results in both parents having to work.

How wonderful to know that an older brother or sister is supporting you and the saints in their prayers.

A church member in her late 70s became increasingly hard of hearing, but was adept at using the internet. She took on the role of missionary-prayer liaison, finding out from missionaries their needs for prayer and passing them on to the fellowship.

In the same way an older church member could obtain prayer requests from younger members and pass them to a group of seniors who would commit to pray for them. Young people have many prayer needs, from examinations to career choices to relationships to money and all stops in between!

There is the biblical example that reverberates throughout history of Moses, Aaron and Hur, all octogenarians, praying whilst up the mountain while Joshua (the youngster) was fighting the Amalekites (Exodus 17:816). Moses makes it clear it was the older men's prayers that really won the battle.

Also, Daniel, then aged 80, praying with all his

heart for Israel and the resulting visit by the angel
Gabriel with the powerful prophetic word.

> *'As for me, far be it from me that I should sin
> against the Lord by failing to pray for you.'*
>
> **—1 Samuel 12:23**

> *'Daniel ... got down on his knees three times a day
> and prayed and gave thanks before his God,'*
>
> **—Daniel 6:10**

Some Scriptural injunctions about good works

LOOKING AFTER OTHERS

> *'Religion that is pure and undefiled before God the
> Father, is this: to visit orphans and widows in their
> affliction, and to keep oneself unstained from the world.'*
>
> **—James 1:27**

> *'Bear one another's burdens, and so fulfill the law
> of Christ'*
>
> **—Galatians 6:2**

> *'We who are strong have an obligation to bear with
> the failings of the weak, and not to please ourselves.'*
>
> **—Romans 15:1**

'Let each of you look not only to his own interests, but also to the interests of others.'

—Philippians 2:4

ENCOURAGING AND STRENGTHENING OTHERS

'Therefore encourage one another and build one another up, just as you are doing'

—1 Thessalonians 5:11

'Do not neglect to do good and to share what you have, for such sacrifices are pleasing to God,'

—Hebrews 13:16

SERVING THE CHURCH

'And God has appointed in the church first apostles, second prophets, third teachers, then miracles, then gifts of healing, helping, administrating, and various kinds of tongues.'

—1 Corinthians 12:28

'In the same way, let your light shine before others, so that they may see your good works and give glory to your Father who is in heaven.'

—Matthew 5:16

'And there was a prophetess, Anna, the daughter of Phanuel, of the tribe of Asher.

She was advanced in years, having lived with her husband seven years from when she was a virgin, and then as a widow until she was eighty-four. She did not depart from the temple, worshiping with fasting and prayer night and day.

And coming up at that very hour she began to give thanks to God and to speak of him to all who were waiting for the redemption of Jerusalem.'

—Luke 2: 36,27

At 84 years of age, Mrs Anna (nee) Phanuel was fulfilling God's purpose for her. She had the great blessing of seeing the Christ child with her own eyes, and the privilege of telling others that He had arrived.

RECOGNISING THE HINDRANCES AND THE HELPS

Things that hinder

a. *Social attitudes towards older people*, which can limit expectations of effectiveness and usefulness.

b. *Lack of self worth:* a low view of one's abilities inhibits a sense of purpose.

c. *Church practices and attitude* – where older people are sometimes overlooked in favour of the young.

d. *Acceptance of perceived limitations with age* – sometimes this means believing the enemy of our souls, who wants to diminish our effectiveness by undermining our confidence.

e. *Personal characteristics* that the Holy Spirit hasn't been allowed to deal with, that can be strong in old age, such as impatience, an attitude of entitlement, self-pity, ingratitude, self-righteousness, argumentativeness, always being right, and others.

Note: Physical or mental frailty is not a hindrance to being useful in old age.

Things that help

a. First and foremost examining your attitude, recognising what is unhelpful and changing it. Psalm 139 says, *'Search my heart Oh Lord, and see if there be any hurtful thing in me.'*

Proverbs 23:7 says: *'For as a man thinks in his heart, so is he'* in other words, we are shaped by our thoughts.

b. When churches encourage and involve their older people, giving opportunities to witness and serve.

c. Whilst accepting that they have to adapt

to the physical limitations of aging, older people can be blessed and invigorated by being reminded that they are part of God's plan, are valuable, and have significant roles and duties.

d. Trusting in God to lead and strengthen: Philippians 4:13 says: 'I can do all this through Him who gives me strength' and in Chapter 1 of the same book, verses 19-20, we're reminded of the ongoing potential of the work of the Holy Spirit: 'For I know that this will turn out for my deliverance through your prayer and the supply of the Spirit of Jesus Christ, according to my earnest expectation and hope that in nothing I shall be ashamed, but with all boldness, as always, so now also Christ will be magnified in my body, whether by life or by death.'

e. Also, recognising the supremacy of Christ, Philippians 2;13 says: 'for it is God who is at work in you, both to will and to work for His good pleasure.'

f. Taking care not to become complacent, and always pressing on 'toward the goal for the

prize of the upward call of God in Christ
Jesus.' Philippians 3:14

'I being on the way, the Lord led me ...'

—Genesis 24:27

THE KEY TO USEFULNESS

Essential Scripture verses that illustrate the most important thing of all

There are many promises for old age in the Bible. Just a few of them are:

'With a long life I will satisfy him and let him see My salvation.'

—Psalm 91:16

'Therefore we do not lose heart. Even though our outward man is perishing, yet the inward man is being renewed day by day.'

—2 Corinthians 4:16

'A grey head is a crown of glory; It is found in the way of righteousness.'

—Proverbs 16:35

But the key is to be rooted and grounded in Christ; to be able to serve others not from a position of intellectual assent to a set of principles, but out of a personal relationship with the Lord.

'Those who are planted in the house of the LORD shall flourish in the courts of our God. They shall still bear fruit in old age; they shall be fresh and flourishing, to declare that the LORD is upright; He is my rock, and there is no unrighteousness in Him.'

—Psalm 92:13-15

'We do not want you to become lazy, but to imitate those who through faith and patience inherit what has been promised.'

—Hebrews 6:12

Examples of older people serving

The Bible is full of examples of older people serving. We've already heard about the prophetess

Anna (Luke 2) and of course we can all recall Job, whose unshaking faithfulness is a constant source of encouragement. Inspiration also comes from Moses, Noah and Zechariah. And Caleb and Joshua, both proclaiming their age and at the same time saying, *'Give me this mountain!'* Joshua 14

A modern example could be Charles Wesley, a man who came to Christ at the age of 31 and continued to serve until his death at 81 years old. Charles didn't just compose over 6,000 of the world's most loved and enduring hymns, but was also an active evangelist.

In a similar vein, Francis Schaeffer didn't write his first book until he was 46, and had a profound impact across the world through his writings and speaking until his death at the age of 72. In fact, just one year before his death, he was conferred with an honorary Doctor of Laws degree by the Simon Greenleaf School of Law (Anaheim, California) in recognition of his apologetic writings and ministry.

Then there are the likes of Martyn Lloyd-Jones and John Blanchard. Lloyd-Jones published the first of many books at 59, and is still one of the most popular and influential Christian thinkers through books and recordings. Blanchard is still preaching, teaching and writing at over 80, and has had in excess of 18 million publications sold in over 60 languages.

In our housing and care homes our 'pilgrims', some in their late 90s and 100s hold fund raising events for missionaries and pray regularly for them and for others. Even people with dementia will sometimes 'break through' and pray. Their prayers help shape events and hearts.

God has opportunities for older people right up to the time He calls them Home. Jean came into our extra care housing in Yorkshire when she was in her nineties. She said she hadn't expected to still be making friends at the age of 96! She enjoyed life at Royd Court very much. Eventually she became very frail and the time came when she seemed to be stepping into Glory. When the District end-of-life team arrived, Jean held the nurse's hand and asked her, 'Do you know where you will go when you die?' The nurse's answer was non-committal, so Jean told her, 'I know where I'm going because I've asked Jesus Christ to be my Saviour. You need to go to church and do the same.'

David and his wife Betty led a full life in commerce and in missionary work until, in their old age, Betty developed dementia and they both moved into a care home in South Wales. It's a popular, Christian care home, but David wanted to strengthen its Christian ethos by forming a regular 'Friends' group, drawn from local evangelical churches, who would visit and encourage the believers and witness to unbelievers. He emailed leaders of the churches, sharing his vision and inviting them to an event launching the initiative. He was in charge of all the arrangements, including inviting speakers. It was a great success and the home now benefits from all kinds of help, practical and spiritual.

David is 93 years old. In 2011 he wrote a book of their lives called, 'The Little Things,' published by 'Onwards and Upwards'. A review by the Rev'd James (Penarth) described it as 'adventure of discovering and doing God's will ... of disappointment and fulfilment but supremely a story of perseverance by the Grace of God.' Betty and David are pictured on the back cover.

These are examples of those who are, as the Amplified Bible puts it:

'[Growing in grace] they shall still bring forth fruit in old age; they shall be full of sap [of spiritual vitality] and [rich in the] verdure [of trust, love, and contentment].'

—Psalm 92:14

'What gain has the worker from his toil? I have seen the business that God has given to the children of man to be busy with.

He has made everything beautiful in its time.

Also, he has put eternity into man's heart, yet so that he cannot find out what God has done from the beginning to the end.

I perceived that there is nothing better for them than to be joyful and to do good as long as they live;

also that everyone should eat and drink and take pleasure in all his toil – this is God's gift to man'

—Ecclesiastes 3: 9-13

EMPOWERING AND ENGAGING OLDER PEOPLE

The Pilgrims' Friend Society was founded in 1807, and has over 200 years practical, 'hands-on' experience and understanding of older people.

We are frequently invited to take workshops and talks in churches and other organisations, and are always pleased to be able to share our experience and knowledge.

Working with a host church, we arrange conferences in different regions throughout the year. We also attend national exhibitions, such as Christian Resources and New Wine.

Our speakers include experts in their field, both from PFS and from others in different specialisms. All are evangelical Christians and all speak from practical experience as well as academic knowledge.

We are constantly refining and developing our workshops and seminars. We keep up to date with clinical research on old age and dementia, and we also monitor participants' feedback for issues arising.

Typical of feedback comments from 'Developing Usefulness in Old Age' is a retired school teacher. She told us:

'I've been active all my life but at the age of 70 thought I was past it. I thought it would be downhill on the way now. But what I've heard has shown me that God still has plans for me, and I'm going forward looking for what He puts in my path to do.'

On page 33 is a list of some of the seminar topics we are asked to address.

TALKS AND SEMINARS

1. Making a truly dementia friendly church

2. Dementia – practical and spiritual insights

3. Dementia – the support and help that churches can give

4. Early dementia and the vital circles of support

5. Visiting people with dementia

6. Giving effective support to family caregivers

7. Empowering and engaging older people

8. Caregivers – how to care for yourselves

9. Ministering in care homes

10. Dealing with loneliness

11. How to prepare for a great old age

12. Developing your talents and gifting after retirement

13. Empowering older people

14. Caring for elderly parents and other relatives

ORGANISATIONS
THAT CAN HELP:

Here is a selection of organisations that are geared up to helping older people.

1. **Age UK** (formerly Age Concern and Help The Aged) – the UK's largest charity working with and for older people, with links to local branches.

    Tel: 0800 169 6565;

    website: www.ageuk.org.uk

2. **Shared Lives** - the UK network for family-based and small-scale ways of supporting adults. Shared Lives used to be known as Adult Placement.

    website: www.sharedlivesplus.org.uk/

3. **Alzheimer's Society** – the UK's leading care and research charity for people with dementia and their carers.

    Tel: 0845 300 0336;

    website: www.alzheimers.org.uk

4. **Care Quality Commission** – website shows rating for UK care homes.

    Tel: 03000 616161

    website: www.cqc.org.uk

5. **Carer's Allowance Unit** – part of Department of Work and Pensions, giving advice on the Carer's Allowance, the main state benefit for carers.

    Tel: 0845 608 4321;

    Text Phone: 0845 604 5312

    website: www.direct.gov.uk/carers-allowance

6. **Carers' Christian Fellowship** – offers mutual support, sharing and prayer.

    Tel: 023 8028 3270;

    website: www.carerschristianfellowship.org

7. **Carers UK** – offers support with caring for carers.

    Tel: 0808 808 7777;

    website: www.carersuk.org

8. **Brunel Care** (incorporating Dementia Care Trust) – offers accommodation, health care, counselling and other assistance, to prolong an independent lifestyle.

    Tel: 0117 914 4200;

    website: www.brunelcare.org.uk

9. **Dementia UK** – offering practical advice and emotional
    support to people affected by dementia through fully
    trained Admiral Nurses

    Tel: 020 7874 7200;

    website: www.dementiauk.org

    Admiral Nursing Direct: 0845 257 9406

10. **Dementia Web (formerly DISC)** – an all-age
    dementia information resource for the UK, providing
    information about other related services across the UK

    Tel: 0845 120 4048;

    website: www.dementiaweb.org.uk

11. **Tourism For All** – charity specialising in accessible
    holiday and respite services for older and disabled
    people and their carers (helps make tourism
    welcoming to all).

    Tel: 0845 124 9971;

    website: www.tourismforall.org.uk

12. **Office of the Public Guardian**

    – helps with planning for one's future.

    Tel: 0300 456 0300;

    website: www.publicguardian.gov.uk

13. **PARCHE** – Pastoral Action in Residential Care Homes for the Elderly; training for church teams.

    Tel: 01323 438527;

    website: www.parche.org.uk

14. **Parish Nursing Ministries UK** – whole person health care through the local church.

    Tel: 01788 817904;

    website: www.parishnursing.org.uk

15. **The Frontotemporal Dementia Support Group** (incorporating Pick's Disease Support Group) – caring for people with Frontotemporal dementia, with regional links.

    website: www.ftdsg.org

16. **Relatives and Residents Association** – information about residential care and help if things go wrong.

    Tel: 020 7359 8136;

    website: www.relres.org

17. **Contented Dementia Trust (formerly SPECAL)** – dementia charity providing courses, services and advice. Is known best for its themed approach to care.

    website: www.contenteddementiatrust.org

18. **Carers Trust (formerly Princess Royal Trust and Crossroads Care)** – works to improve carers' services and helps carers make their needs and voices heard.

    Tel: 0844 800 4361

    website: www.carers.org

19. **Independent Age** – advice and information on home care, care homes, going into hospital and related issues.

    Tel: 0845 262 1863

    website: www.independentage.org

20. **AT Dementia** – Information on assistive technology for people with dementia.

    Tel: 0116 257 5017

    website: atdementia.org.uk

21. **Guideposts Trust** – provides direct services to people with dementia, their families and carers, to help them make the best choice for care services.

    Tel: 01993 772886;

    website: guidepoststrust.org.uk

22. **Alzheimer's Research UK** – provides information on the different types of dementia, their symptoms and the treatments available to help.

    Tel: 01223 843899

    website: www.alzheimersresearchuk.org

International

23. **Age International** - helps older people in developing
    countries by reducing poverty, improving health,
    protecting rights and responding to emergencies.

    website: https://www.ageinternational.org.uk/